MULTIPLE
SCLEROSIS

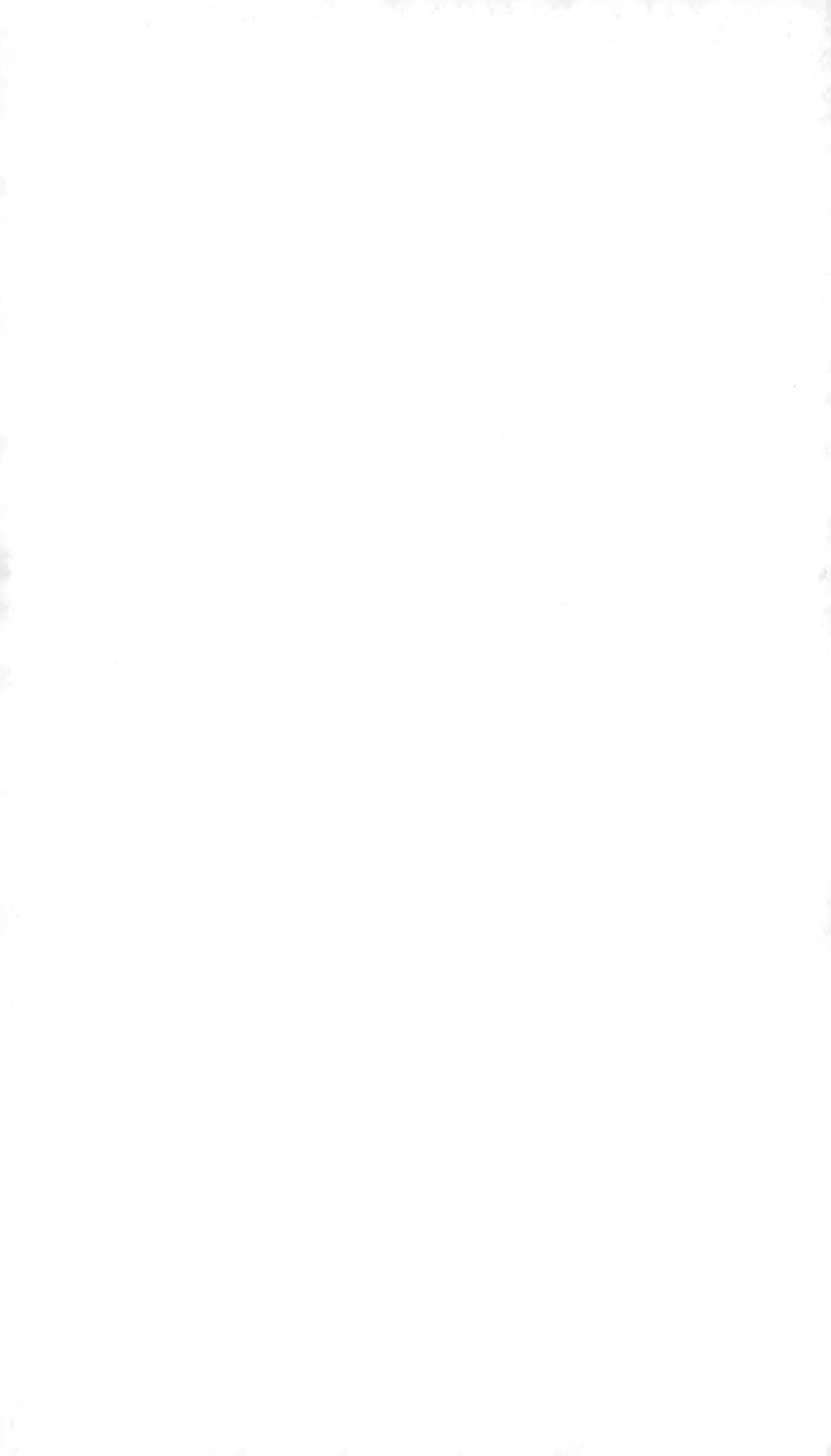

MULTIPLE SCLEROSIS

On the path from cause to cure

SUSAN A NORBERG

ISBN-13: 9781522935391
ISBN-10: 1522935398

DEDICATION

I am so grateful for all the support I get. I am truly blessed to be surrounded by such good people. And to my husband Jim, where would I be without you? Your compassion and patience get me through each day.

TABLE OF CONTENTS

INTRODUCTION

It has been many years since being diagnosed, and what began with a slight limp progressed to a wheelchair in a matter of a few years.

There is so much more information available today than when I was first diagnosed, especially concerning the importance of diet, movement, and outlook. Due to the fact that all medicines have side effects, it behooves one to take a look into potential alternatives. Even among many in the mainstream medical community, there has been a growing acceptance of herbal remedies. A big part of what I have come to learn is that we are all unique. Each one of us has not gotten here due to the same cause. So it only stands to reason that our remedies for healing may be as varied as our causes.

To all the readers of this book, I hope I am able to offer some insight into what might be the answer to many of the questions you have had in your own personal journey. I am not a doctor nor am I in the medical profession, I am simply sharing my own path with you on the decisions I made. So if you are considering any of the following suggestions, please seek advice from an expert, and beware, herbal remedies may interact with prescriptions you may be taking.

Chapter 1

SYMPTOMS

It was January of 1989 when I had such a bad case of the flu that I was barely able to walk, spending most of my time bed ridden for at least two weeks. When the worst of the sickness had passed, I returned to my daily routines of working, bowling, and taking care of my two boys ages eight and six. Although I survived the flu and returned to health, I noticed I was walking with a slight limp. Of course I told myself this would eventually go away. This one symptom would just take a little longer.

In spite of the slight limp, which was probably more noticeable to me than to others, I returned to the bowling league. It was around this time that I began to feel a tingling in my feet. I had recently bought a new pair of sneakers. They felt a bit snug and I wondered if that numbing pins and needles sensation was due to a lack of circulation. I became more and more concerned when it was no longer just a tingling sensation I was feeling, but a loss of balance. I would pick up the 12 pound bowling ball, and as I walked toward the pins swinging my arm, I found it increasingly difficult to walk straight to the point where I was afraid I might fall over.

Since being diagnosed with multiple sclerosis, I have looked back at my life and tried to determine what I may have done that would have contributed to the onset of this disease. I know I was under a lot of stress at this time in my life. More than my usual stresses of work, raising two children, and the everyday managing the budget, juggling of money and schedules. I was very active. Weight was never an issue I was always thin. I wish now looking back I had a healthier diet. I had (should say have) a sweet tooth. A chocoholic and addicted to carbs. Oh yes, and I shouldn't leave out, knocking back a few beers here and there. I don't believe there has been a genetic connection to the disease. At least not in my family. I'm not aware of anybody that's any relation to me now or in the past who has had multiple sclerosis. So here I was, sure it must be something that I had brought about through my lifestyle.

It was in July of 1989, when I woke one morning with the symptom I simply could not ignore. As I got out of bed I nearly fell to the floor. My legs would barely move. They felt extremely heavy as if there were weights tied to my ankles. It was at this point I was no longer able to remain in denial. I knew I had to go seek out help, and this is where my journey began.

Chapter 2

MEDICAL DIAGNOSIS

It seems almost ironic to end up at a walk-in clinic. I couldn't walk. I clung to my husband's arm while limping. Nothing much came from that visit. A few pages of blood work, a suggestion that I see a neurologist, and a bill.

I had been fairly healthy and had not seen a doctor in many years. It took a few months for me to find a physician willing to see me. It must've been August or September when I finally arranged an appointment with a local doctor who ordered blood work and proceeded to test my reflexes. They were supersensitive and I kicked the doctor startling him. He had never seen such reflexes and I remember him exclaiming how he wished there were interns there to observe my reactions to his little hammer. He had his receptionist set up an appointment (I believe it was in October 1989), for me to see a neurologist.

The neurologist ran tests. From BAER (I think it was called this) and EEG, to three MRIs. It was with the MRI of the brain, that he finally found what he believed was the problem and set up an appointment for me to come in to discuss the test results.

It's interesting how our minds work. I can't remember what I had for dinner last night, but there are pivotal moments that could be less than a minute long, and occurred many years ago, that I can still recall in my mind with such clarity. One of those moments occurred in the doctor's office the moment I was forced to face the truth of what was behind all of the symptoms that had now been progressing for months. It was now January 1990. The folder with my test results sat on the desk in front of the doctor. I watched as he opened it. I saw the pages of his writing and what I can still remember to this day, was him telling me that I have chronic progressive multiple sclerosis, and in my mind's eye on the bottom of the page, I can still see him writing the letters MS and circling it with his pen. I wondered if that was intentional. That if I saw him write it down it might somehow help me accept the unacceptable. He asked if I had any questions but I had trouble thinking of any. I do remember asking him how long he thought I might live. He said he didn't know, it could even be 20 years. He proceeded to write a prescription for baclofen.

P. S. I am in my 26th year

Chapter 3

PRAYER AND MEDITATION

I have always believed in God. Somehow it seems easier to believe that there is an intelligence behind all this madness than to believe that all of this is totally random. I remember praying for a miracle, asking God if he would cure me. I thought about it a moment later and realized how selfish that sounded. There were probably millions of people with multiple sclerosis, that God should only heal me? I changed my prayer at that moment and I asked God to please help to find a cure for the sickness so that no one should have to suffer with this.

I believe it was November 1989 when I was scheduled for my first MRI. I followed all of the directions, making sure I did not have any metal on me. I changed into the gown they provided and climbed onto the (whatever you call it), that slid me into the MRI machine. It didn't go well. I had my first panic attack. I was so disappointed in myself.

I was raised Catholic and kept a rosary in a small box on the night stand beside my bed. The next morning the children were in school and my husband had gone to work. I was alone in my bedroom praying my rosary. I ended my prayers saying "please lead me, guide me, show me." I remember that morning feeling particularly sad and expressed it in the sudden release of tears. There was a book that I had gotten autographed by George Anderson (a psychic who I will be discussing in the next chapter) that along with his autograph wrote a lovely message. In it he referred to St. Philomena. I didn't know anything about her so I researched and found information along with a prayer specifically for St. Philomena, then folded the paper and left it inside the book. I felt so hopeless. For the first time in my life I was facing a situation where there was nothing I could do to help myself, and nothing anyone else could do to help me, no medicine could cure me, and I felt strangely alone in my feelings and frightened of my unknown future. I took out, from his book, the folded piece of paper with the prayer to St. Philomena, it read:

> Prayer to St. Philomena
> Illustrious virgin and martyr St. Philomena behold me kneeling in spirit before the throne on which it has pleased the most Holy Trinity to place thee. Full of confidence in thy protection I beseech thee to intercede for me with God. From the height of thy heavenly country, deign to cast a look upon thy humble servant. Spouse of Jesus Christ, console me in my troubles, strengthen me in my temptations, protect me in the dangers which surround me on every side. Obtain all the graces necessary for me, especially (here mentioning in your particular intentions), and above all, assist me at my death. Amen

I can't recall my particular intention word for word but I do remember asking for the strength to help me get through whatever testing I needed to go through.

I finished my prayer. I laid quiet in a meditative state when the most incredible thing happened. As if someone was whispering in my ear, so clearly in an audible voice I heard the words, "Sometimes things have to get worse before they get better". And in that moment I felt a peace and security I have never felt in my life. A warmth ran through my body. The sadness was replaced with the feeling of hope. I have since thought of this moment of perfect peace, and I have a feeling that this is what I can best describe, as what it must feel like to be one with God.

I've had a few of what I would call my spiritual moments. Occurrences that transcend the norm. Defy explanation. Off the side of my house was a screened porch. On a sunny day, in nice weather, I would enjoy sitting outside in the fresh air. One particular afternoon I thought I might try meditating. I had often tried it but never really seemed to have enough patience to sit quiet and keep my mind still long enough to notice any benefit. Instead I would just sit there thinking of all the things I should be doing. Probably not a good idea. So I thought I might start with a prayer. I asked God "If it is not my time to be healed, is there something I could do to help me feel better"? I closed my eyes and immediately a cartoon appeared in my mind of a man disappearing into a bush. I opened my eyes in reaction to that vision. I closed my eyes once more, and immediately the sight of the bush appeared, only this time with no leaves on it. I dismissed the thought. It made no sense. Some hours passed and then all of a sudden I understood. I understood it was about living food. It was about diet. It was about the importance of vegetables and fruits.

I tested this, purchasing a juice extractor, juicing apples, carrots, celery and just about any concoction of fruits and vegetables available in my refrigerator. There was a definite connection between my diet and my nerves. The vegetables and fruits I had been juicing had a calming effect on my nerves as opposed to the jumpy, tense, uncomfortable feeling I had when I ate too much sugar. So the meditation was the answer to my prayer as to what would help me feel better. The cartoon of the man had devoured the leaves of the plant, and so should I.

So my best advice is to pay attention.

* Pay attention to that song that suddenly pops into your head. This has happened to me occasionally. I can recall once having a difficult time. I prayed about it one morning uncertain of how to handle the situation. As I was walking down the stairs that morning I noticed the song *Let It Be* began playing in my head. I especially remember it ending with the words "There will be an answer, let it be."

* Pay attention to the people that mysteriously show up in your life. I recently broke my leg and I was in the rehab center when the physical therapist came up to me and told me that she had a dream that I was walking. She handed

me a pamphlet from a healthcare facility that focused on nutrition for healing. I also remember when I was first diagnosed with multiple sclerosis the little girl that lived next door came over one day and told me she had a dream that I was walking. I have occasionally had these dreams myself. They give me hope. I know it can be hard, but try to keep a positive outlook, stay hopeful. Which leads me to my next point.

* Pay attention to your dreams. As a matter of fact try asking a question just before you go to sleep, or better yet writing it down. Hopefully if you can remember your dreams come morning, they will include somewhere in the interpretation, an answer to your question. I have had this experience. I retell it in Chapter 7. *The Dentist, The Dream.*

They say when you pray you speak to God, and when you meditate God speaks to you. How true.

Chapter 4

THE PSYCHIC

I moved to my house in 1985. It was around this time I discovered a TV show featuring the psychic George Anderson. He had a live studio audience and would do random readings when he felt prompted by souls that had passed on. He would also take live phone calls and do the same. His accuracy was amazing.

He also offered readings from his home. I felt fortunate when I was finally able to get through his very busy telephone line after many attempts to make an appointment. This would be my first appointment. It was May 1989. I was excited to get the reading, and didn't have to wait very long in his waiting room before he called me in and asked me to take a seat. I brought with me a book he had written (as I mentioned in the previous chapter) entitled *We Don't Die*. I asked for his autograph and he graciously signed

"To Susan,
May the Lord bless you and yours always here and in the hereafter. St. Philomena, refuse not the aid of thy prayers to us that plead for it venerating thy merits.
Sincerely, George Anderson"

It was this autograph I referred to in my moment of despair, when I called on St. Philomena in Chapter 3.

It was four years later in either March or April of 1993 when I was able to get a second appointment. It must have been at least six months before my appointment due to his long waiting list. Although mostly using a wheelchair at this point, I arrived at his home using a walker (as I did for short distances), so it was no surprise to me when he brought up the issue of my health. He picked up a pencil and pad and began scribbling, asking me if I knew specific people living or dead as he threw out familiar names awaiting my acknowledgment. He asked me if my grandparents spoke with an accent. I told him they did. He then proceeded to describe my symptoms from head to toe and finally said to me that I had multiple sclerosis. He told me they were saying I eat way too much sugar (O.K, so I'm still working on that one) that I should eat more fruits and vegetables. He told me they were saying to leave the mainstream medicine and seek alternatives.

He then said "They say you handle it well."

I told him I'm surrounded by really good people.

He said they agreed. That I have a lot of support.

He also told me of other information past and future. It was uncanny how much he already knew about my past, but there was one thing that did not seem likely. He told me I would be going away on a pleasurable form of travel. I said I sincerely doubt that as I am not at all comfortable taking long trips. He told me "no... they say you're going". Well I was proved wrong. One day while out shopping with my husband, we passed a local car dealership and there in the parking lot was a used motorhome. So it was on a whim we decided to stop and take a look. It seemed very well priced and I was thrilled when I managed to get up through the door the couple steps needed. I looked around and I saw possibility. There was a small kitchen, a dining booth, toilet, shower, and all close enough where if I needed to balance myself there was plenty to hold onto. Don't you know we ended up buying it? We had not taken a vacation in so long and after going through it, it seemed absolutely possible that I could be comfortable. So even his unlikely prediction came true.

Continuing on with the reading, he asked me if I knew of Margaret. I said no. He then said Margaret Ann? I said I couldn't think of anyone. He asked if I knew Al. I said yes I did. Al was my husband's father. He told me he would be passing soon, that they were gathering on the other side to greet him as he passes over. This saddened me, even though I knew in my heart he was fighting a losing battle with cancer. I debated with myself whether or not to discuss this with my mother-in-law. I decided to tell her. I figured why would they tell me this information unless they wanted my in-laws to know. I brought up the name Margaret or Margaret Ann. She told me that was his mother's name. One month after my visit to the psychic medium George Anderson, my father-in-law, Al, passed away with Marion's final words to him, "I release you to your mother's arms".

He closed the reading by telling me that someone named Frank, an uncle like figure, was thanking me for my prayers. I told him that he had been a boss in a previous job. He then told me that everyone that came through thanked me for my prayers and was surrounding me with a blue healing light.

I know there are many skeptics. They don't believe that anyone can be contacted by the souls of others who have passed away or perhaps they don't even believe in life after death, but even they might change their mind if they experienced the accuracy of a reading from a true medium.

And so I took with me that day, the two most important pieces of health information from George Anderson

1. Change of diet and
2. Leave the mainstream medicine and seek alternatives

Chapter 5

EDGAR CAYCE

In my quest seeking alternatives to the mainstream medicine, I decided it was important for me to take myself off of the baclofen. I began taking vitamin supplements, and like I said before, I began making changes in my diet.

Along with the changes I made to my diet, I continued my journey by seeking new alternatives outside the mainstream. I decided to find out what information Edgar Cayce might have said about the treatment, if any, of multiple sclerosis. For those who might not be familiar with Edgar Cayce, he was a very popular psychic living from 1877 through 1945. He is considered the father of holistic medicine by many, and also known as the 'sleeping prophet'. He would lay down and go into a trance. He had a stenographer who would present him with information such as the person's name, the date, and their address. He would then diagnose the problem and give specific details on what they could do to remedy their sickness or problem. He did this for 44 years and has the largest record of readings of any psychic.

I sent away for all the information I could get from the Edgar Cayce library regarding multiple sclerosis and later with the motorhome, took a vacation to Virginia Beach where we visited his research center. But the information I received was more complicated than I expected. You see there wasn't one answer or solution to healing. Each reading was individual. Everyone wasn't given the same response. But in spite of the differences in the readings as to the exact advice he would offer, there seemed to be three recurring remedies that were consistent.

* Wet cell battery
* Massage
* Diet

The wet cell battery was a weak battery made with a specific solution (specific to the individual whose reading it was), then attached to the body with wires at various locations on the body depending upon each individual. Often the lack of gold was mentioned as the cause of the imbalance in hormones, never to be ingested, but instead added by vibration through the use of the wet cell battery. (I don't really understand this). The gold seemed to be the most prominent of solutions mentioned in his readings however depending on the reading for the individual, there were other solutions such as iodine tri-chloride, Silver Nitrate, spirits of camphor etc., but mostly gold chloride.

His readings concerning massage, were as varied as his solutions for the wet cell appliance. Depending upon the individual reading, the oils could be anything from olive oil, peanut oil, melted lanolin, oil of sassafras to a combination of oils. He would often recommend the massages be carried out immediately after the use of the wet cell appliance.

He was a very spiritual man and often referred to the Bible, citing certain passages to be read while carrying out these therapies.

Concerning the diet, most readings indicated alkaline diet, non-constipating, and low in fat. Other foods that were stressed were foods with B vitamins. He said the vitamin B aided the nervous system. As far as meats went he recommended

* Seafood
* Liver
* Wild game
* Foul

These were to be broiled and not fried. He mentioned seafood specifically for the iodine. He said iodine had an effect on all the endocrine glands not only the thyroid. He said to stay away from pork. He also mentioned various vegetables depending on the individuals.

The causes or reasons for the disease, as always varied from individual to individual however most frequently revolved around the liver and its ability to make other glands in the body function properly, some sort of liver thyroid balance. He also mentioned problems with assimilation of food, by that they assume he meant problems with digestion. A lack of gold or other metals or minerals which would cause an imbalance in a hormone produced by the liver. Seeing as the liver is not a gland, science and medicine of that day could not have understood the meaning of this reading.

There is so much information, and so much of it is so specific to each individual that it makes it very difficult to try to come up with one universal treatment for everyone. He also states that it would typically take anywhere from three to seven years before someone is cured. So although I did start to try to make changes in my lifestyle, I remained skeptical as to whether I would ever be successful following any one specific reading from the Edgar Cayce's files.

I remember bringing this information with me on my routine checkup with my neurologist. I mentioned to him that according to Edgar Cayce a part of the problem was a lack of a particular metal or gold. He seemed very interested and asked who Edgar Cayce was and where he got this information. He said he always felt it had something to do with the metals. I told him Edgar Cayce was a psychic and this was done through personal readings for people with multiple sclerosis. Oh well, that was the end of that. He had no more interest in pursuing further information along that vein. Another one of those moments that I can still recall, was when my neurologist pushed the Edgar Casey file containing the cure for multiple sclerosis back across his desk toward me. Did I detect a slight eye roll? Me thinks so.

Chapter 6

THE GOOD, THE BAD, THE UGLY BACTERIA

From my meditation on my porch, to my visit with psychic George Anderson, to the readings by Edgar Cayce, there ran a common thread. Each one pointed to diet as an essential factor affecting my multiple sclerosis. All three stressed the importance of fruits and vegetables. Added to that was the admonishment by my grandmother through the psychic George Anderson that I ate way too much sugar.

Understanding the digestive system and its effect on the body became very important in understanding just how critical foods are to our health. I can't point to one particular source along the way that I could reference and acknowledge, but I finally understand how absolutely damaging sugar is to our health.

We have within our digestive system good bacteria and bad bacteria. It is extremely important that we maintain a level of good bacteria higher than that of bad bacteria. Unfortunately sugar feeds the bad bacteria. The bad bacteria then grows and grows in increasing numbers over time, outnumbering the good bacteria that is essential to the digestion of our food. We then crave more and more sugar due to the high level of bad bacteria feeding on it. The digestive system now overwhelmingly consisting of bad bacteria, causes an imbalance in the ratio of good bacteria to bad bacteria. When our digestive system becomes out of balance and overwhelmed with bad bacteria we are susceptible to contracting what is known as a leaky gut. Then the toxic bacteria can leak into our blood system and begin affecting the cells in our body causing all kinds of disease. This may be a likely cause of much of the autoimmune disease. Also, a portion of the conversion of the thyroid hormone takes place here. You will see later why this is so important.

Another large problem is the overwhelming amount of antibiotics dispensed by many in the medical community to their patients. Of course they should be taken when necessary, unfortunately there are many instances when they are administered as a precaution. Even our food. The meats we eat, if not organically fed, contain antibiotics. Regardless of the reason for receiving antibiotics, they are not only killing the bad bacteria but also the good bacteria. Therefore make sure you are always replenishing your supply of good bacteria by introducing probiotics at the same time to help prevent an imbalance of too much bad bacteria. Probiotics should be part of the daily diet.

Chapter 7

THE DENTIST, THE DREAM

I no longer remember what year, what network, or who it was being interviewed that day on the news. I do remember a young woman discussing an incredible discovery she made upon having her amalgam fillings removed by her dentist. Prior to that visit she was having symptoms common to the symptoms related to multiple sclerosis. One of those symptoms was with her difficulty in walking. Amazingly after having her fillings removed she returned to her former state of health. The symptoms simply went away.

I found this very interesting especially after reading the Edgar Cayce files on multiple sclerosis. Some of his readings in which the people were diagnosed with multiple sclerosis, according to him, were actually misdiagnosed. He found, in his trancelike state, that they actually had mercury poisoning. That mercury poisoning has symptoms similar to multiple sclerosis. The amalgam fillings used by dentists contained mercury.

I called my dentist's office to make an appointment to have my fillings removed. I told the receptionist the reason for the appointment. She told me that she would have the dentist return my call when he got a chance because she had never had such a request. It wasn't long before he returned my call. He told me the chances were very slim the fillings were the reason for my symptoms. To remove them might actually just cause more problems, and that he didn't recommend me proceeding down that path.

I retold the story of the woman on the news and how she had regained her health by having her fillings removed. He didn't seem very impressed.

He hesitated then said, "Do you know what the odds are that your fillings are actually causing your symptoms?"

I remember I said to him, "If it were you, and you knew you had a one in a million chance you would walk again… would you do it?"

I remember the silence at the other end of the phone, a sigh, then he responded.

"Come in… we'll talk."

My dental appointment was rapidly approaching and I hadn't come to a firm decision whether or not to go ahead and remove the fillings. I have often felt at odds with the medical community and it always becomes a very difficult decision on which path to follow. Do you go with your own gut trusting your intuition, or take the advice and recommendations of the medical experts. Who do you trust more? I vacillated on the pros and cons and decided to take it to a higher source. At night before going to sleep, I prayed for guidance. That night I had a dream.

In the dream I was walking along the sidewalk in front of a local strip mall. My husband came walking toward me. It appeared he had been at the drugstore to get my medicine. He says to me, "You're not going to believe who the pharmacist was."

I asked, "Who?"

He said, "George Anderson."

I was really surprised by that, then he told me, "and he said to tell you it's not AM it's AU."

That's when the dream ended.

When I awoke, I remembered the dream and I understood exactly what it meant. When I had gone to the psychic George Anderson he told me to leave the mainstream and seek alternatives.

I realized the importance of the symbols in the dream. The AM referred to the amalgam fillings I wanted removed, that contained mercury. The AU referred to gold, the symbol on the periodic chart of elements. So the message was clear. The dream was answered. I was to continue pursuing the alternative by listening to the psychics. The lack of gold was often mentioned in the Edgar Cayce files as a problematic factor in the cause of multiple sclerosis.

Chapter 8

PNEUMONIA AND THYROID SICK

Over the years I learned a very tough lesson. Do not get sick. Each time I get sick, I feel as though I never totally heal. From that first flu in 1989 when I began limping, to every sickness since, I have found I am left with a diminished effect of my abilities.

Between Christmas of 2014 and Easter of 2015 I had two bouts of pneumonia. The second episode of pneumonia was so serious that I was intubated and quite frankly don't have much recollection of this period of time. One good thing that came out of it, was that I was finally diagnosed with a thyroid condition. I know it may sound crazy that I'm considering this a good thing, but because of this diagnosis I began researching the thyroid where I discovered a lot of useful information leading to my understanding of what is most likely another large piece of the puzzle of the cause of multiple sclerosis.

For a long time I had noticed my hands and feet were always very cold. My fingernails were very brittle and my skin was very dry and easily cut. My hair seemed to be thinning, however, it wasn't very noticeable as I had fairly thick hair. I began taking my temperature. It frightened me when I found it falling well below the normal 98.6°. This concerned me and by checking online, there seemed to be two causes, one hypothermia (when someone's body temperature is dropping quicker than it can recoup itself, like in a prolonged cold environment), and the other hypothyroid (a problem with low thyroid hormone). I had my thyroid level checked and according to the doctor my TSH (thyroid stimulating hormone) level fell within the normal range.

My second trip to the hospital with pneumonia was when I was told I needed medicine for my thyroid. So this diagnosis of a thyroid condition felt like good news when I left the hospital with a prescription for levothyroxine. Finally something would be done to alleviate the symptoms. Or so I thought. Within six weeks of being home from the hospital, my hair began to fall out. I was still cold, but now even colder as I was near bald. I remained bedridden severely weakened from the pneumonia. Thankfully I was able to locate a nurse practitioner that would make house calls and provide me with any blood tests needed.

I found a wonderful book by author Suzy Cohen. I highly recommend this book for everyone. She gives a comprehensive explanation of how the thyroid works. What I discovered was that the pituitary gland at the base of the brain receives a message from your hypothalamus to produce the hormone TSH (thyroid stimulating hormone). A TSH test is what is commonly used by doctors to test if your thyroid is healthy. The thyroid then releases a hormone called T4. Besides what T4 does for the body as far as detoxification, it also needs to be converted into a T3 hormone. Apparently every cell in our body requires the T3 hormone to function properly. (The T stands for thyroid, the 3 for the number of receptors.) This T3 hormone affects every aspect of our lives from body temperature, heart rate etc. If the cells in our bodies are to survive it is essential for them to receive this hormone.

So how does the hormone T4 get converted into the T3 needed by every single cell in your body? The conversion of the T4 into the T3 mostly takes place in the liver (although it will also take place in the brain and during digestion and in other organs and the cells themselves.) The T3 is then transported to the cells through the blood by using iodide or other essential minerals. And remember it is only the T3 that is able to be used by the cells (which also have 3 receptors) not the T4. The T4 must be converted to T3. If there is too much T3, the reverse T3 (rT3) shuts the door on the cell, blocking it from entering. Too much rT3 blocking the T3 from entering, and you have the beginning of unhealthy cells. The liver is producing too much reverse (r T3) could very well be the problem considering it is the organ where most of the conversion takes place from T4 to T3 and rT3. Other problems that can occur that block the T3 from getting to the cells, can be everyday toxins like the fluoride in our toothpaste, and other chemicals that poison our system whether taken internally, or those present in our environment.

So why so much discussion about the thyroid? Because it's important to understand what's going on with our cells in our body and how it affects our health, and why this is most probably a very large reason for what is causing autoimmune diseases. The thyroid getting sent a message to release the T4 hormone. The T4 hormone making its way to the liver where it is then converted to the necessary balance between the T3 and rT3. The T3 being transported through the blood via specific minerals. The minerals provided through the digestive system. The health of the digestive system dependent upon nutritional diet and proper balance of bacteria.

It is so much more in depth so many great suggestions in the book about the thyroid. The tests she (Suze Cohen) recommends. The foods to eat, to the supplements to take. She discusses the different causes of this problem that may be potential problems such as the Epstein-Barr virus, or even if you had your appendix removed. Like I said, I highly recommend reading it.

In my particular case, after being released from the hospital (still weakened from the pneumonia), my nurse practitioner ordered blood tests, the first of which were slightly improved in comparison to those blood tests formally taken by the hospital. There were still some disappointing readings and so more blood tests followed.

These tests were of much more concern. There was concern about my liver, and a very high TSH count. This was very confusing because the results indicated I was hyperthyroid (too much thyroid hormone) while the symptoms appeared I was hypothyroid (too little thyroid hormone). I couldn't run the comb through my hair without a large amount of it remaining in the comb with each stroke. More and more hair went down the drain with each wash. The symptoms simply did not reflect the results of the blood tests.

Chapter 9

MY LIVER, MY THYROID, AND ME

It was the fact that the worst of my hair falling out, occurred six weeks after being released from the hospital, that made me link the hair loss to the prescription of levothyroxine prescribed by the hospital. I remembered a previous conversation with my nurse practitioner about hormone medicine, when she told me it takes six weeks to kick in. I decided to take myself off the medicine. I found out that Levothyroxine is a T4 medicine, and what I believe was happening was that I didn't have a thyroid problem at all. My thyroid was perfectly capable of producing T4. I did not need T4, what I needed was T3. I needed the T3 hormone that is produced by the liver. Therefore the addition of the T4 medicine (levothyroxine), to the T4 my thyroid was already putting out, created a high reading making it appear as though I was hyperthyroid.

The abnormality of my liver was very concerning. I remembered my sister mentioning that she had a problem with her liver. It was a nonalcoholic form of cirrhosis. This condition, known as fatty liver disease, is becoming more and more common in the general population. I called to see how she was, and mentioned that I too was having an issue with my liver according to my blood tests. She then told me that hers was cured. Her doctor wrote her a script for a chelate and recommended she take selenium. Besides being available as a supplement, foods such as nuts, fish and whole grains are often high in selenium.

So I believe the problem lies in the conversion of the hormone itself. Like I mentioned before, the main organ in which the conversion of the T4 into the T3 takes place, is in the liver. When the T4 gets to the liver it has the ability to produce T3 or rT3 (reverse T3). Remember the rT3 keeps the proper balance of your hormone so that you don't build up too much T3 and it does so by blocking the access of the T3 into the cell. Therefore too much of the rT3 is bad for you. The more you have the worse you will feel for it lowers your thyroid activity, hence the symptoms of loss of hair, brittle nails, etc.

So you're probably wondering what all of this has to do with multiple sclerosis. Well this has to do with all autoimmune disease one of which is multiple sclerosis. The weakening of the cells in our bodies due to their inability to get a hormone they need for them to exist and be healthy. In the case of multiple sclerosis, this damage occurs in the nervous system.

Chapter 10

THE STRESS FACTOR

Conversion of the thyroid hormone also takes place within the cells. Apparently stress can be such a significant factor in the inability for the cells to convert the thyroid hormone to the T3 needed, I should therefore address that here. Now this is something that I feel in particular pertained to me as a partial cause of the onset of the multiple sclerosis. And I have no doubt that Suzy Cohen is right. This is a common problem in much of the population. The role that stress plays in our lives on a daily basis and the effect it could have on our health. In particular our adrenal gland. I believe this may have been mentioned in the Edgar Casey files in one or more of his readings.

For anyone interested in looking into the workings of the adrenal glands, there are very informative YouTube videos I found by a chiropractor Dr. John Bergman. He gives very interesting detailed information on how our bodies work. He discusses the adrenal glands that pump out the hormone cortisol and the balance that takes place, between the thyroid hormone and the adrenal hormone cortisol. Apparently the cortisol is the hormone that the body uses in times of stress. It is the fight or flight hormone that kicks in to protect us in an emergency. It is meant in these times only and not for prolonged stress. When we are stressed and the cortisol takes over, the thyroid hormone is suppressed. In other words, when the cortisol gets pumped up the thyroid hormone gets pushed down. When the stress is over, the cortisol goes back down and the thyroid hormone goes back up to normal. When we live in the prolonged state of stress and the cortisol is up too long, and the thyroid remains depressed for too long, we end up with what is known as adrenal fatigue. The adrenal gland is not meant to constantly be in that stressful state for an extended period of time.

Suzy Cohen recommends testing the adrenal gland before you even bother trying to correct the thyroid. That there is no point in taking any medication for the thyroid if you don't have the adrenal gland functioning properly. Who knows, this might be a part of the reason why Edgar Casey puts such a large emphasis on massage as a big contributor towards healing of multiple sclerosis. Relaxing the body. Making sure your glands are producing the proper amount of thyroid hormone and not in the state of stress creating too much cortisol which in turn would be suppressing the thyroid hormone..

Chapter 11

RELAPSE/REMIT
WHAT IF...

It has been over 25 years since being diagnosed with chronic progressive multiple sclerosis. I barely remember what it was like to feel normal. Howerver, the majority of people diagnosed with multiple sclerosis (probably 80 to 90%) have relapsing/remitting MS, often then in later years followed by a secondary progressive form of MS.

I'm going to speculate now about this form of MS.

What if...
You spent the summer swimming in a built-in pool full of chlorine, quenching your thirst by drinking lots and lots of chlorinated water from the tap. Sprayed pesticides on those annoying insects, fleas, ticks, even termites and ants. What if then this causes an abundance of chemicals with three receptors preventing the T3 hormone access to the cells.

What if...
You went off that great diet you were on and binged on sugary desserts. Messed up the balance of good and bad bacteria, pouring toxins into your bloodsream.

What if...
You drank or smoked. Maybe you were a little too happy. Maybe you were little too sad. Maybe you're even taking prescription medications. Caused some problems with your liver throwing the T3 and rT3 ratio out of balance.

What if...
You suddenly fell under a lot of stress. Pressures at work. Pressures at home. You end up with a bad case of adrenal fatigue.

Now

What if...
You suddenly had a relapse of multiple sclerosis. You no longer feel well. So you stop swimming in the pool, you know you should be eating better and you're too sick to go to work. Maybe the relapse is so bad it leaves you bed ridden.

Time passes. And NOW *what if...*
the chlorine from the pool water leaves your system. The very chlorine with the three receptors that was depriving your cells of the T3 hormone

What if... The relapse scares you into eating healthy. You know you've been eating too much sugar and carbohydrates. That leaky gut stops sending toxins to the cells.

And *what if...* Resting at home away from your job or whatever problem situation caused stress has finally subsided, correcting the balance of cortisol to T4 thyroid hormone.

Then maybe… Your relapse was exactly the thing that brought about the remission. That by *your choices* you are able to tip the balance one way or another between relapsing and remission.

It would be interesting to record those periods of time. Keep a diary of foods and activities. You just might find a pattern of the events or foods responsible for the occurrences of those times you relapse. If you can isolate what might be at the root of these occurrences, then through the simple act of avoidance you just might be able to stay symptom-free. It's just a thought. But

WHAT IF...

Chapter 12

FROM CAUSE TO CURE

I have been led to the answer of a prayer that I prayed many years ago. I questioned why me and what should I do? I prayed that there might be a cure. I've been led down a path through the meditations, the psychic visits, doctor visits, the books I've read, and the people I've met along the way, and I feel as though I now understand the cause.

For me, I feel I owe it to a combination of causes. I owe it to my many years of a bad diet, a long bout of stress, liver problems, toxins like fluoride, pesticides, and who knows whatever else.

So where do you start? What caused your MS in the first place? Who knows? We each have our own unique reasons for contracting this disease. Get tested and find out which of any of these problems may be causing the destruction of your nerve cells. Perhaps you too have a liver problem. Perhaps you have specific vitamin, mineral, or hormonal deficiencies. Maybe you are under a lot of stress. The important point is that given the proper nutrients, exercise and relaxation, our bodies have the ability to heal themselves. So get tested, check for deficiencies. Maybe the easiest place to start is your diet. Work on what is causing the inability to assimilate (digest) food properly. The leaky gut. This then can cause a lack of essential minerals and other necessary nutrients for the transportation of the T3 hormone essential for our cells. Edgar Cayce recommends an alkaline diet. An alkaline diet consists of mostly fruits and vegetables. This sort of diet can help prevent arthritis and other problems too. And again over and over I hear the most destructive of food is the sugar we eat.

And so it is so important to include probiotics. I don't believe there is ever a problem of too much good bacteria, however there is definitely a problem when you have too much bad bacteria. It is toxic. It contributes to, and slowly begins the decline in our cells abilities to function properly, until eventually they cease to function.

A common deficiency among people with multiple sclerosis is vitamin D. Why is it that people living closest to the equator do not get multiple sclerosis? Could it be we spend less time outdoors? Or because there is less daylight year round? Could it be because the UVB rays reach them year-round, while north of a specific latitude the UVB rays only reach that part of the world from April through October? Probably all of the above. Rather than risk skin cancer by over exposure to the sun, perhaps boost the vitamin D through supplements. I have personally begun taking 5000 IUs of vitamin D3.

After reading this book on the thyroid, I looked back at the beginning of my journey. I pulled out my Edgar Cayce file and began rereading his description of the cause of multiple sclerosis. How the lack of particular minerals and or gold created an imbalance of particular hormones produced by the liver. Again of course in those days, during his lifetime, it would've seemed absurd according to the scientific community, for the liver to produce a hormone, being that there was no glands in the liver. But now we know. We know that the thyroid produces T4. We know the T4 once in the liver produces either T3 or reverse T3. (Thank you Suze Cohen). So even though the liver is not a gland it is actually producing hormones. We know there needs to be a proper balance of these hormones in order to maintain healthy cells in our bodies. For these hormones feed every single cell in our body and are essential for our health and our lives. Is your liver creating too much rT3? The reverse T3 (r T3) will block the cells, preventing the T3 from being able to access the cells. It would be worth having the ratio of these levels tested. (I know it sounds redundant, it's worth repeating)

So now I am understanding the causes, and I am hopeful I will be heading down the path to a cure. I understand from the Edgar Cayce readings that this is a process and a slow one for he did say it would take 3 to 7 years. And I understand why. I can remember seeing Deepak Chopra on the Oprah Winfrey show discussing our body's ability to reproduce new cells. He discussed how it took(I believe he said) approximately seven years for every single cell in our body to reproduce itself, how in that amount of time we are actually physically not the same person we were seven years ago.

We are what we eat. In Edgar Cayce's readings he points out specific foods to eat and in the Thyroid

Healthy book by Suzy Cohen, again certain foods plus essential vitamins and other supplements. In my own meditation I can remember the odd vision that came to me pointing me to an alkaline diet of plant life.

There is a connection to the importance of the assimilation (digestion) of essential nutrients and their part in transporting the T3 to the cells. Making sure I have plenty of probiotics in my diet. The importance of the seafood (I don't eat much fish due to mercury, however I have switched to using Himalayan salt) due to the iodine it provides and the other minerals.

I've stopped using toothpaste with fluoride. Many of these chemicals that end in IDE apparently contained three receptors as does iodide (the mineral with the three receptors that is actually needed by the T3). Unfortunately the T3 needed by our cells (again worth repeating) doesn't know the difference between the toxic chemicals with three receptors and the iodide.

The health of the liver is extremely important in making sure it is functioning properly so that it can produce and maintain the proper hormonal balance between T3 to r T3. See if you can have a blood test that could give you the ratio between the T3 and the rT3. Also have your adrenal levels checked. Again I have to highly recommend Suzy Cohen's book Thyroid Healthy, in which she gives detailed explanations of why so many people are not feeling well, along with suggestions of what tests to take and what nutritional remedies are recommended.

Try things like selenium, phosphatidylcholine, milk thistle, things that are cleansing to the liver. Change your toothpaste to an all-natural choice without fluoride. Certain drugs prevent the conversion of the T4 into the T3. There is so much to know. I understand now why Edgar Casey's readings were so specific to each individual. We are all unique in our particular needs and or deficiencies.

Fresh air and sunlight for Vitamin D, all things in moderation. Pray, meditate, exercise, keep those muscles toned, for who knows, in 3 to 7 years, you may be needing them on your road to health. Oh yes and don't forget, PAY ATTENTION.

Do your best to stay stress-free. Relax get a massage. I can directly pinpoint the beginning of my symptoms coinciding with a very stressful time in my life. I remember Dr. Oz discussing that our DNA is like those shoestring ends, and that stress has the ability to make the DNA fray just like the ends of the shoelaces when they lose their plastic tips. I only wish I knew over 25 years ago what I know now. Those words I heard so many years ago from the audible voice following my prayer. "Sometimes things have to get worse before they get better," give me hope that the worst is now behind me and the healing will start as I begin implementing these changes to my life.

So if you're seeking an alternative to the mainstream in healing, you might want to immerse yourself in a holistic approach in dealing with this disease. Involve your body, mind, and spirit. There will be bad days no doubt, but try to stay positive. Our bodies believe what our mind tells it. Eating right, thinking right, and having faith, will help us to create change at a cellular level. It will just take time.

Chapter 13

SUMMARY

Spirit:

* Pray
* Meditate
* Dreams...Ask questions...look for answers
* Listen to uplifting music

Mind:

* Get a hobby. Do something creative. It's a drug free antidepressant. We all need something to look forward to. It can uplift your spirit while entertaining your mind.:
* Think Positive
* Pay attention
* Interact with others with positive outlook or similar interests.

Body:

* Get your adrenal levels tested
* Get lots of sleep (I've got to work on this)
* Take Probiotics (So important)
* Buy Organic Food
* Beware of toxic chemicals like chlorine and pesticides
* Make Changes such as eating and juicing fresh fruits and vegetables, replacing your butter with coconut oil, and replacing all-purpose

flour with almond flour or other gluten-free flour, beware of sugar

* Change Your Toothpaste Eliminate fluoride
* Exercise, even your eyes
* take supplements like magnesium and vitamin D, COQ10, etc. (get lab tests and research benefits and hazards of the different vitamins and minerals)
* Cleanse Your Liver with supplements such as phosphatidylcholine, milk thistle etc.
* Quit smoking, alcohol, and coffee. Coffee depletes the Selenium which Converts T4 into T3
* Maintain an Alkaline Diet
* Drink lots of water
* Try Acupuncture (works well for many)
* Since all medication has side effects, if you are taking a prescription find out what essential metals, minerals and vitamins may need supplementing (if you must need medicine)
* Get tested for your T3 and rT3 ratio. (Hopefully you be able to find a healthcare professional who will be able to help you facilitate any testing necessary)
* Please, Please, Please... Read the book *Thyroid Healthy* by Suzy Cohen. There is so much important information with a holistic approach and guidelines for testing. She recommends testing on the adrenal glands as an

important requirement especially for people with autoimmune disease, also provides valuable information as to which herbal supplements are helpful

* *if interested contact the Edgar Casey research Center in Virginia Beach for information regarding his readings and the wet cell battery (this could be difficult as I previously mentioned, the ingredients were specific to each individual reading)

Like I said in the beginning, I am not a doctor, nor am I in the health profession, I am only here to share my journey with others that are on a similar path and seeking answers. Edgar Casey said the cause of multiple sclerosis was due to poor assimilation (digestion ....leaky gut?) causing the lack of a particular metal or mineral, (depending on the person) that creates an imbalance of a hormone produced by the liver (the balance between the T3 and the rT3?)

Edgar Casey said it would take 3 to 7 years. Why? I suppose it's because that's how long it takes to regenerate new cells? I know 3 to 7 years sounds like a long time. But replacing the sick cells with new healthy cells is essential. It just takes time. What else do we have to do that is more important?

It's been 26 years since I started down this path seeking answers. I wonder sometimes, if I would still be here had I stayed on the medicine originally prescribed. I am sharing this information with everyone that might also be interested in seeking healing through a holistic approach. It's funny how the very source from what many would consider controversial readings of a psychic from the distant past, would eventually connect me to the science of today.

As I said, I am by no means an expert, and the information I am providing in this book, is a simplified and condensed version of the very complex workings of the human body. So if you find your current treatment isn't helping, and you decide to seek an alternative holistic approach, I'm hoping this information will help you. At least it might be a good place to start.

To all of you, I wish the best of luck on your path to a cure.

EPILOGUE

Since implementing some of these ideas, and having taken myself off my thyroid medicine (levothyroxine) I have already noticed improvement. Not only has my hair stopped falling out, but I have noticed significant growth. My fingernails are no longer brittle and my skin is not as dry and frail as it was months ago.

I have been taking phosphatidylcholine now for over one month and my blood test on my liver has greatly improved.

I realize I've got a long way to go. This didn't happen overnight. It's been over 26 years in the making. What lies ahead? Only time will tell.

REFERENCES:

Thyroid Healthy
By Suzy Cohen

YouTube
Chiropractor Dr. John Bergman

Research Bulletin
Multiple Sclerosis
* Edgar Cayce Foundation
67th & Atlantic
Virginia Beach, Virginia 23451

The Edgar Cayce A.R.E. Website offers an list of
foods detailing which are alkaline and which are
acidic. Great resource.

For information about the psychic medium George Anderson, he has a website
www.georgeanderson.com
To order this book visit
http://www.mscause2cure.com
www.createspace.com/5851541
also
Available at Amazon.com and other retail outlets